LAYLA JEAN

What To Do When Breathwork Doesn't Work

Tips and tricks to get results with breathwork.

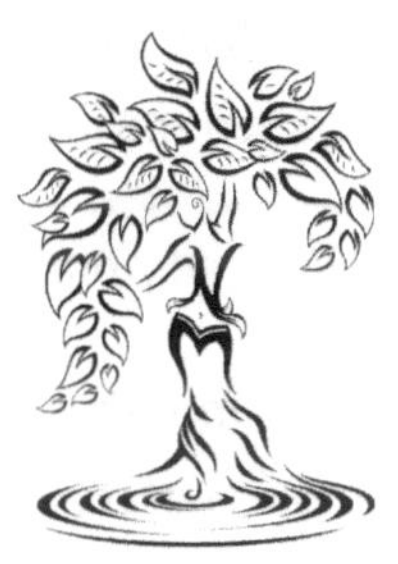

This book was professionally typeset on Reedsy.
Find out more at reedsy.com

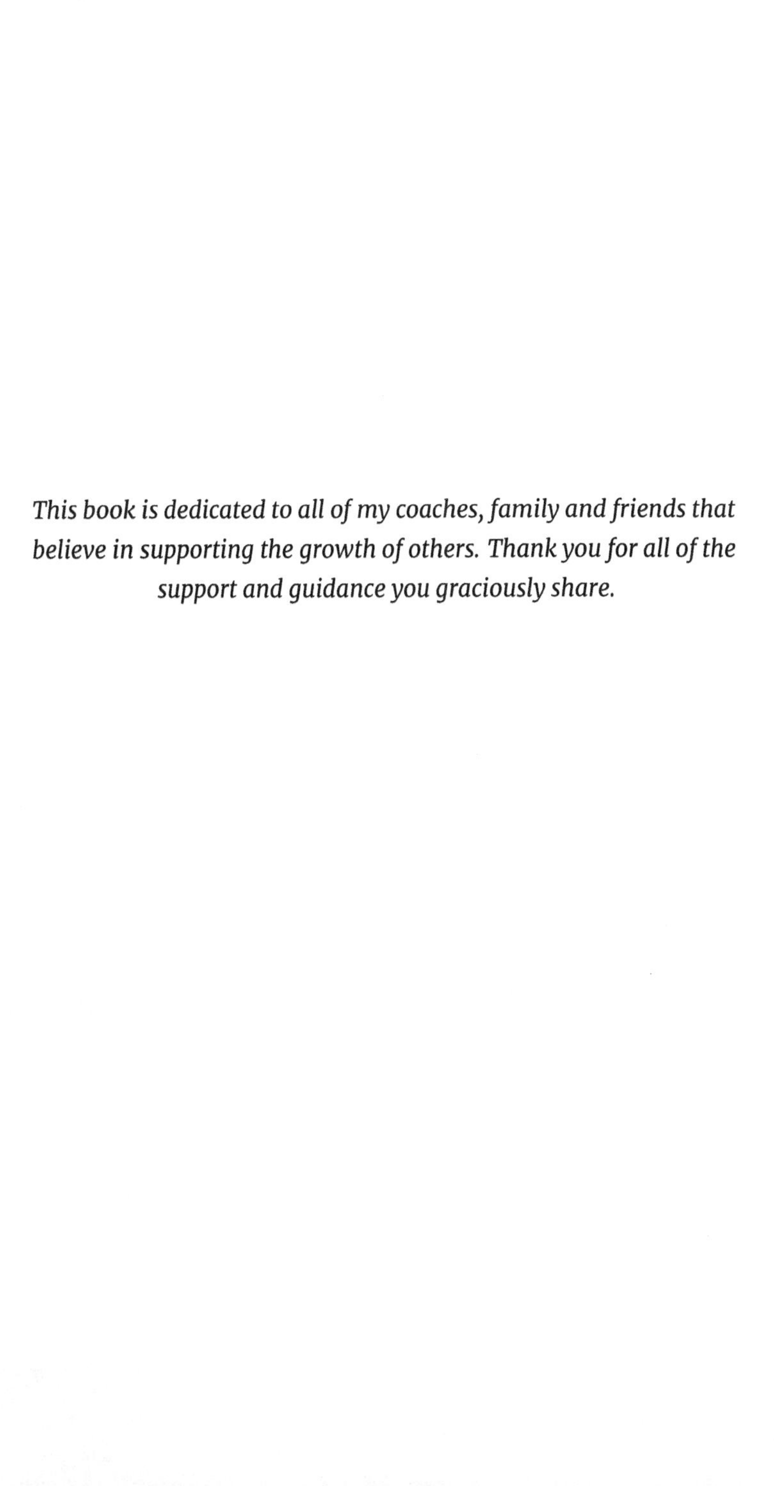

This book is dedicated to all of my coaches, family and friends that believe in supporting the growth of others. Thank you for all of the support and guidance you graciously share.

Contents

Preface

Have you ever been told to calm down, take a chill pill, or everything is just fine when you were under pressure, and everything wasn't just fine? How about "just breathe!" I can tell you when that happened to me in the past it wasn't a pretty picture. It can be downright frustrating. People who say things like that to others under stress or panic truly mean well, but probably have no idea how unhelpful that can be to hear.

Hi, my name is Layla Jean and I have been there before. My guess is if you picked this book up you have too and are looking for solutions to better manage stress when everything you have tried in the past hasn't worked for you.

After years of frustration, developing symptoms of pain, overwhelm and illness I finally took matters into my own hands. I took steps to learn more about what options are out there for people like us. I spent years studying and exploring until I could finally understand what was behind the scenes in my mind and body keeping me from being able to relax. That is when I was able to develop a plan that I could use whenever I needed to embody the art of breathwork.

While the suggestions in this book have helped countless people it is very important to understand the benefits and possible challenges you may experience.

Please consult your medical provider to ensure breathwork

is suitable for you. Breathing exercises may present a risk of harm for people with certain medical and or neurological conditions, including epilepsy, cardiovascular issues, anxiety and PTSD or people who are pregnant.

Please feel free to share this book with your provider for their approval.

Breathwork is truly an art form. We may not see ourselves as talented masters in the arts but guess what. I am here to tell you it is totally possible to learn and develop your skills when you have the right support and information available. It isn't your fault that breathwork hasn't been easy or is not working for you up to this point. It isn't abnormal that you find it difficult, impossible, or even irritating. That is why I am writing this book. I feel strongly there is a gap in the learning process of using breathwork as a tool for stress management. I spent so much time spinning my wheels looking for solutions I could embody when my mind was too busy to let me relax enough to take the time to breathe. This book is meant to offer you a simplified version detailing the highlights of what you need to know to be able to use and receive the benefits of the vast world of breathwork. I promise breathwork is not a sham. It can open you up to so much more rest and freedom if you are willing to take the time to practice some of the suggested ideas in this book. Too get the most benefit from this book I recommend reading it all the way through and imagine doing each recommendation before going into application mode. Feel free to playfully explore each breath pattern and notice if it resonates positively in your body. Notice what makes sense to you and your circumstances. Because we are all so unique.

You have permission to make your experience of exploration, better understanding and practice exactly what feels best for you.

So get your favorite beverage, Find a relaxing place to sit, and let's get started on this new pathway to stress relief through breathwork.

1

Why isn't breathwork working?

First off let's explore why breathwork may not be working. Most likely when you have tried in the past to lay down in a relaxed space and close your eyes while focusing on your breathwork you have found the mind racing, problem solving, planning, rehashing that last conversation that was stressful or awkward, organizing the next day, wondering when you will feel different, how long is this going to take, I really need to do those other chores, I don't think this is helping, and finally I don't have time for this.

All these thoughts flying through your mind at lightning speed keeping you distracted from the mission happen because the information we needed to know wasn't available or we haven't put the time into understand the process. We may have viewed breathwork as time consuming, silly, or to new age for our taste. But more so we probably haven't taken the time to recognize the current behaviors we have are because of how we see the world. You see, most likely we are full of anxiety from all our past experiences or traumas. Big or small as they might be it doesn't matter. It is the lens we have looked through and the way we have developed the habits, ideas, and even possibly disabilities we currently function inside of. If I look back over time I can now see how I have spent years being a perfectionist, trying to please people, trying to be liked, to fit in, to be in control of everything and everyone around me. Can you relate? We have been trained and have rehearsed this way of life for years. We may have been told this is how to get ahead, be successful, be worthy or have value. The rat race of doing this and doing that is a real thing, but thankfully it is between the ears, and we can learn to choose differently. We can say hold on; this way of thinking isn't serving me anymore. It's plain and simple and isn't working and is causing more harm than good.

Here is some good news. NONE OF IT IS YOUR FAULT, BUT IT IS YOUR RESPONSIBILITY. There are solutions and the stress patterns we perform in can end if we want them to. Simplified, it doesn't matter what the trauma or life experiences were in the past, it is simply important to recognize them and see if there is a lesson you can learn from them and release the painful memory that keeps you stuck in a world of stress. We don't have to rehash the past over and over anymore. We don't have to carry the heavy burden anymore. We can simply ask "what was I supposed to learn from that experience?" Embrace that lesson. Quite possibly the lesson is that the past situation wasn't even your fault. That it wasn't something you could control. Or maybe you had a hand in it and it was an opportunity to see what doesn't work. Could it be it was teaching you a better way to live. Have gratitude that whatever we go through has the power to make us stronger, wiser, and more empathetic. We can choose a better way of thinking and free ourselves from the burden of carrying painful memories and trying to function with the weight of it on our shoulders. If we don't choose to let it go we never will. There is so much power in being brave and bold enough to explore letting go of the negative past and embracing the lessons of embodying a new way of thinking.

While this book is meant to be a quick handbook guide to use breathwork to manage stress, I do highly recommend reflecting on the previous paragraphs and exploring the idea of finding a personal coach or counselor to learn the best approach for your unique healing exploration.

Later in this book I list breathing techniques that can be used hand in hand with council and coaches and can truly help us free ourselves more quickly from burden bearing our past wounds or even the burdens of other people we care about. When we are finally ready to let it all go and enjoy the teachings of the trials. If you have found your way to this book you most definitely are ready for a change. Especially when there are so many more joyful things to give our attention to. Understanding the mental health component is one of the most rewarding and helpful steps we can take on our journey to being able to embody the stress relief practices of breathwork. Living life free of the past pain will give you more joy and that joy will continue to snowball into other areas of your life in amazing and unexpected ways. It is such a beautiful experience ans so worth the time and commitment each of us needs to put in at the start. As we grow it all becomes so much easier and we will most likely crave the freedom breathwork can offer.

Other possible things that are keeping us from success in using

breathwork may be:

● Time limitations. Needing to learn how to prioritize yourself so you can fill your cup. Or the belief that it takes long intervals of time to have success.

● Personal beliefs. Just the statement "I can't" playing in your head and out of your mouth is enough to make it impossible. We must stop and take thoughts like that captive and retrain our thinking patterns to align with our desire for better health.

● Too many outside distractions. Who hasn't been there before. Learning to say no or please wait can free you from overwhelm. I find it helpful to give my full attention to people for the first 10 minutes (especially children) and then explain you need the next time frame of your choosing to take care of yourself. And then you can come back to them. You get to choose how much time you need to take care of yourself and it may be different day to day. But, do make sure to keep your promise to them after you keep your promise to yourself. It builds trust and understanding as well as self-competence for both parties.

●Understanding the impact of other people's anxiety is crucial; we often unknowingly absorb their emotional signals like antennas. Learning breathwork techniques can be invaluable in such situations. Through practice, we gain the ability to differentiate between our own energy and that of others, allowing us to filter what we internalize. This realization is profound; it empowers us to recognize that much of what we feel or react to isn't inherently ours.

- Personally, acknowledging this truth enabled me to reclaim control over my peace and happiness. Practices like breathwork can be incredibly helpful in grounding ourselves and creating a sense of inner calm amidst external chaos. By focusing on our breath, we can center ourselves in the present moment and cultivate awareness of our own internal state. This awareness allows us to recognize when we're being influenced by external energies and helps us choose how to respond rather than react automatically.

- Needing boundaries and the practice of self-care are also important aspects of managing the impact of other people's emotions. It's okay to prioritize our own well-being and to take steps to protect our energy when necessary. By recognizing that not everything we feel belongs to us, we can reclaim our power and cultivate greater peace and happiness in our lives.

● Missing information."Just breathe" is often the message we are told and we hear it from the well meaning friend exactly and the most irritating time when they think we need it the most. However, we need it most before we get to the point of crisis. If breathwork isn't trained and practiced, we won't be able to engage it successfully because we will be too distracted and overwhelmed. We are often taught it is supposed to be easy. No one tells us that the ease comes with previous practice that makes it familiar and natural. We often think we need to do it for hours on end and are not taught how valuable a minute of mindful breathing can be. In the next chapter we will look at more helpful insights to becoming successful with breathwork to reduce stress and provide a better overall state of wellness.

● Fear of the woo-woo. Will I be seen as ungrounded and silly for trying something that is unique or seems unusual? What will the "committee of they" think if I make noise when I breathe in public? Fear of woo-woo is the inner skeptic trying to keep the ego safe. It is dismissing other important and valid ways of living that have proven over time to have massive benefits. Ask a Lamaze instructor how woo-woo breathing techniques are. They will be able to set you straight on that topic. Fact is, breathwork is scientifically proven to provide profound benefits.

A Place For Notes:

2

Steps to take now to learn how to embody breathwork

Breathwork is a type of work. It takes time to develop the skill just like any new habit. One of the best points of view I hope you can embrace is that it is a practice. So be kind and patient with yourself. We can build this new habit by setting simple and easy goals as you begin your practice. At the end of each section feel free to take time to write or journal your experience as you try things out. As you continue to grow in your practice it is a great idea to continue to write your experience down. What and how you feel? What changes do you notice? What did you like or dislike? and How do you think it will change your day? How will you know if you are successful? are some suggested ideas to write about to get you started.

Here are some suggestions of first goals and action steps to begin with.

● Make it your daily habit before getting out of bed in the morning or even possibly before you even open your eyes to take three big and meaningful breaths, keeping a smile on your face while you do it. Try to set other specific times to add a breath or two to a daily habit you do already. Before brushing your teeth or when you first step in the shower. There is plenty scientific proof out there showing linking a new habit to a current habit will increase the success ratio of maintaining the new desired habit. Practice a breath pattern as you complete a small task like while cleaning something or walking across the room to get something. Keep it simple, short and sweet.

● When you take a moment to be mindful of your breath, compliment yourself for taking action. And when you forget and remember later tell yourself "It is okay not to be perfect at this. You are getting better already" Then take a few satisfying breaths. Don't be hard on yourself. Treat yourself like your own personal best friend.

● Celebrate your success and notice how you feel when you made the best choice you could in your practice. Really take the time to feel how empowered you feel. See if you can notice a change in your smile or sense of pride that you are winning over what used to be more challenging or impossible. When we embrace the successes, even the tiny ones, we are creating new neural pathways in our brain, and it is setting us up for even more success with less effort.

● Remember breathwork doesn't need to be a 30 plus minute activity. It can be as simple as taking a single mindful breath. Mindfulness is the key. Stay in tuned with the sound of the breath. Pick a pattern of breathing that serves you the most in the situation you are in. We will talk more about that in chapter

3.

● Be willing to make some noise. Breathwork works best when you can hear it. Are you feeling shy? I remember when it used to be very difficult for me to make any sound in public settings. If you find yourself in this situation, a helpful mindset is "I deserve to take up space and it's okay to be heard." I used to also tell myself when I was in a group setting that my sounds of breathing helps others feel safe and encourages others in their practice. It kind of became a simple act of service that I could perform as a gift to others. Start by telling yourself this type of mantra when you are alone in your practice. Then when it is time to be bold and brave and make some noise in a public setting it will be easier. I promise it will get easier the more consistent and accepting you can be when you breath with purpose. In fact you will probably even notice more benefits of stress relief sooner when you allow the sounds of the breathwork to vibrate through your body and out the nose and mouth.

● Make it BIG. Feel the whole body expand like a balloon. Notice where the air goes as you breath in. Does it sit in the upper chest and shoulders? Does the rib cage expand in 360 degrees or only in the front? Does the belly expand? Notice how complete the exhale can be. Making the breath big, full and complete in and out will develop new healthier ways of functioning at a cellular level and bring relief to the whole body. It will also shorten the time it takes for new muscle memory to develop and help maintain a better way of breathing. Remember, If you feel like making noise do it. Let the body know you are listening and give it the release it wants. That noise may even be a holler, shout or growl. It doesn't matter what the sound is. It matters that you are responding to what your body is asking for. It is a good thing. I attribute it to building the trust with in yourself that you will take care of you first.

One of the first things I like to do when I want to practice breathing for a period of time is prepare my environment. Here are my favorite recommendations.

● Create a space you want to be in. Make sure you can control the elements around you. Sounds, temperature, smell, and amount of light are things you may want to consider. Have a favorite comfortable chair, a mat with pillows or cushions. Make sure to have a blanket nearby. Whatever helps you feel comfortable and safe. Make it a place you want to be and show yourself gratitude and kindness in that space. Literally thank yourself for showing up and giving your body a moment to embody peace. If you are worried you may fall asleep feel free to set a timer that will wake you when it is time to go to your next activity. Make sure you are not hard on yourself if you fall asleep during a practice. Celebrate your body got what it needed at that moment and stay encouraged for next time.

● Turn on some music. Be sure it doesn't have lyrics unless it is a guided breathing recording with background music. We don't want the lyrics because it is easy to become distracted and want to sing along to our favorite melodies. I enjoy finding meditative music and guided breathing tracks on my favorite music app. Here are some helpful basic facts. You can put the Hz or emotion in the search bar of your favorite music app to serve your needs in that particular practice. This can be fun to explore what works for you and what you aren't so sure of.

- Binaural beats in the theta of 4 to 8 Hz are linked to reduced anxiety, relaxation, meditation and creativity.
- Binaural beats in the alpha frequencies of 8 to 13 Hz are great for relaxation, positivity, and decreased anxiety.
- 40 Hz beta binaural is a great place to start to increase focus on your practice.
- Frequencies in 432 Hz promote connection and grounding, healing.
- 528 Hz promotes love, peace, and overall wellness.

As you feel more comfortable exploring how you feel in specific parts of your body you can try the below frequencies. I will use one over the other if I feel a heaviness, irritation, or uneasiness in a particular spot and I will choose a corresponding frequency to help give attention to the area in unrest.

- 963 Hz Crown - Located at the top of head - Wisdom, personal connection, and purpose.
- 852 Hz Pineal gland - between the eyes - looking for more clarity, intuition. and understanding.
- 741 Hz Throat - Having a hard time speaking up?
- 639 Hz Heart - Right in between the ribs - Peace, love relationships, release of anxiousness.
- 528 Hz Solar Plexus - In the soft area under the breastbone - better instincts, clarity, and strength.
- 417 Hz Sacral - Located between the hips - creativity and pleasure.
- 396 Hz Root - Located at the base of the spine - stability, safety, connection with nature.

Notice the area of the body you are using the corresponding sound for and imagine your breath filling the space and exhaling out the stress. Imagine the space aligned and vibrating with joyful energy.

Many music and meditation guides are labeled as to what frequency it is using and for what purpose. If you are not sure I would recommend typing in the search bar what you are looking for from the list above. Make sure to take time to reflect on your experience and how you feel. Remember to celebrate your efforts. Notice what feels different. Reflecting will make it easier to continue coming back to your practice in the near future.

⬤ Turn on some mood lighting. Here are some suggestions for colors and the effects they are known for to enhance moods.

- Red: light for calm, playful, strengthening, confidence, vitality.
- Blue: relaxed focus, safety, trustworthiness, communication, effectiveness.
- Green: Soothe emotions, creativity, peace, balance, healing.
- Yellow: Action, motivation, warmth, positive self-esteem, creativity, eating
- Violet: optimism, positivity, wisdom, reflective, peacefulness

Don't be afraid to let the colors rotate or change one into the other. That can be a really nice choice when you are not sure what color you would prefer. Or you are feeling really good and just like the flow.

⬤ Use headphones or ear plugs. Whether to listen to your music or guided breathwork program or to block out distractions. I also find using headphones or earplugs helps me hear my breathing pattern better. This can also help keep the mind on the breathing pattern and strength I am practicing. Learning the sound of your breath as it resonates through your body is also a great way to get more comfortable when you are in a public setting and practicing mindful breathing. It can even help you develop that inner trust we talked about earlier. Just keep focusing on the sound of your breath. In and out.

⬤ Imagery Is another great way to actively get the mind focused on your goals. It can trick your brain into a secondary task that helps you run the program in your mind for mindful breathing. Think of your favorite place and see how comfortable that place is. Imagine smelling your favorite smell. Fresh cut grass, the ocean, coffee, your favorite flower, BBQ or grilling over a campfire. Whatever it is, imagine how it makes you feel and ground yourself in that sense. Imagine tasting your favorite food or beverage and playing with the idea of the flavor twirling in your mouth. Feel how it feels to be satisfied. With each breath in and out, pick a new flavor, smell, or place. Be creative and let go of the ideas of right and wrong. Decide to roll with your breath.

⬤ Using touch. This is one of my favorite techniques to use. There are programs out there that teach techniques like tapping. They are fantastic programs, but for the purpose of simplicity we will explore an even simpler technique called acting on intuition. Notice what part of you wants touch and how. For example, I find it very supportive to gently rub my fingers together and feel each groove of my finger tip. Sometimes I feel like I should tap my forehead in between my eyes. Another favorite thing I do is to gently massage behind my ears or the joint of the jaw with both hands or rub circles on my tummy. The goal isn't to do this right and not wrong, it is to pay attention to what your body is telling you and giving yourself the attention you are asking for. It could be anything, as long as you keep inhaling and exhaling with intention. Let the inhales fill all 360 degrees of your lungs. Let the exhales be loud through an open mouth and complete.

● Close your eyes and focus on how the body feels in the expansion of the inhale and in the contraction of the exhale. If you choose to keep the eyes open, try to relax the line of vision and put your attention to the peripheral vision to relax the eye's gaze and dilate the eye. This will help minimize the amount of information your brain needs to process, open up your gaze, and help decrease distractions.

Special Note: *Feel free to move around, wiggle or rock. Do not feel like you have to be perfectly still. If you have an itch, scratch it. If you find movement supportive move.*

● Sign up for sound baths experiences or other breathwork experiences. Community can be very encouraging when you are feeling unsure or nervous. Look for a community lead by a well-recognized guide or someone who you feel safe exploring with. Don't be afraid to ask questions. The coach has spent years practicing and learning in order to be able to lead a group in a meditation practice. They are excited to share what they have learned along the way and delighted that you have an interest in what they are passionate about. Also, how many times has someone asked a teacher a question and you were like "Oh good,

I was wondering about that too." Normalize speaking up and being seen and heard.

A little more to know before beginning a specific breath pattern.
The Science of inhaling through the nose.

Let's explore why we choose to inhale through the nose and exhale through the mouth in most of our techniques we will be exploring. We inhale through the nose because it does four very important things.

1. It acts as a filter removing impurities from the air and sends it to the sinuses to deal with.

2. The nose acts as a humidifier to moisten the air before it reaches the lungs. Think of a time you were out in the cold dry weather. Maybe even winter in the northern hemisphere. When you inhale through the mouth the air doesn't have the time to warm up before reaching the lungs. This can cause a lot of irritation to the lungs very quickly and you may find yourself coughing and tight. I have at times found it helpful to put a sheet or blanket over my face especially if I am feeling like my nose is dry or irritated. Using a blanket over your head is a great solution if you find your nose is blocked at the time and you need to breathe through the mouth. Let's face it, in some situations any breath we can take is better than not breathing.

3. Another gift that breathing through the nose offers is it slows the inflow of air just enough so the body can balance the level of CO2 with the intake of the oxygen. This is a very cool scientific exploration if you have the time but for

the purpose of the book we will keep it very simple. We have been taught CO2 is the waste product of the breath, but the body actually needs a tiny bit of CO2 with oxygen to help absorb the oxygen into the cells it is feeding to provide energy to that cell.

Just think about what we do when someone is hyperventilating. We have them breath into a paper bag. This is done to help regulate the fact that they are getting too much oxygen putting them in a position of panic because the oxygen they are taking in too fast cannot mix with the CO2 and get into the cells. The body is starving for oxygen. The bag acts as the nose mixing the gasses into the proper amounts so the individual can catch their breath and the whole system calms down because it is being given what it needs to survive.

Did you know too much oxygen can cause dizziness, tingling in extremities, panic, chest pain, swelling in the lungs, ringing in the ear.

Check out what Dr Eric Berg DC has to say in his YouTube video Nose Breathing Amazing Benefits - Why You Should Breathe Through Your Nose. He discusses briefly the condition Hypocapnia. A condition of low CO2 linked to conditions like asthma, COPD, lung infections, panic attacks, anemia, and glycated hemoglobin. This can also turn into a condition called alkalosis: cramping, abdominal pain, laryngeal (throat) spasm, coughing, bronchospasm (lung), tingling lips hands and feet, and tetany). It can even be linked to calcium levels too high or too low. While we may not be Doctors it is still good to know about your body and have some information so we can consult our favorite medical professionals.

Bonus: *Practicing inhaling and exhaling through the nose will also help build nasal and lung capacity.*

A Place For Notes:

3

Favorite go to breath patterns

Three Part Breath or Dirgha Shvasam (Long Breath)

Best for overall wellness and awareness of self, enhancing mood, cognition, relaxation and preparation for focus.

I highly recommend making the 3-part breath your first focus for its powerful ability to support a person in learning body awareness and self appreciation. Other benefits include stress relief effects and overall wellness. Because it is a full body breath that requires attention and awareness to complete in a specific way it is a tool you can use and see the benefits in other areas of life very quickly.

Three Part Breath can be done sitting or my favorite, laying down. It should not be a forceful or pressured inhale. Keeping the breath soft and gentle makes the diaphragm and lungs more able to fill into its fullness and depth. If you are too forceful and push the breath and muscles, you will have a shallow, less effective breath and over all practice. Make sure to keep it slow and complete each part of the breath. When the breath is complete you will have activated the body in this order.

Belly, ribs, and chest on the inhale in that order and on the exhale chest, ribs, belly in that order.

I like to think of it as the waves of a lake or ocean rolling in and out. It has a circular and undulating pattern that is very soothing.

Let's break it down.
Start by practicing each part 10 times by itself before adding it all together as one breath.

● Part one: Get comfortable, place your hand on your belly (abdomen), and inhale filling the belly up as if a balloon is inside. Feel the belly expand and become full. On the exhale let the belly naturally pull inward, noticing the navel pressing to the spine. This action is activating your diaphragm. The muscle right under your lungs that acts like a pump to circulate the air you breath in and out. *It is also one of the many areas in the body where the vagus nerve connects. This nerve is very important in how your bodies organs functions (parasympathetic nervous system). I only bring it up because of how it relates to sensations you may feel in your body. Being able to calm the bodies parasympathetic system may lead to better immune system health and organ health.* Repeat this until it is comfortable and effortless. 7 to 10 times. Once you understand this belly activation part of the breath try practicing part 2 several times by itself and then add part one to part to until that seems to feel easy to do.

● Part two: Place your hands on your rib cage sides (thoracic) and breath in filling up the rib cage (all 365 degrees of it). Notice how expansive the ribcage expands and, on the exhale, feel the muscles between the ribs contract and melt back into the body. If you are sitting down this part of the inhale should feel horizontal through the whole rib cage, back and sides as well as the front. Repeat step two until it feels familiar and effortless. About 7 to 10 breaths. Remember no pressure. Keep it soft and deep. Once you feel successful with part two see if you can add it to part one.

● Part three: Place a hand on the center of the upper chest (clavicle). Inhale into the chest. It should feel like the chest is lifting up vertically. Take your time and explore the different feelings in the body with each inhale and then exhale. Repeat 7 to 10 times.

● Now try to take in the full inhale connecting the three parts: belly, ribs, and chest.

Once you have taken that full inhale, exhale in the reverse order. With the exhale the chest comes down, ribcage contracts gently releasing the air, and belly exhales contracting softly as it empties the breath. One area at a time top to bottom.

This breath can take 10 to 15 seconds to complete a full inhale and exhale softly in the correct order. If you feel heavy or uncomfortable pressure you are most likely breathing in and out too forcefully. Stay soft and relaxed yet full deep and complete.

Nose: Deep soft breath in belly expands, ribs expand, chest lifts.
Nose: Exhale chest falls, ribs contract, belly contracts navel to spine.

Bonus: *It is thought that the deeper you can breathe the deeper* *your understanding of the world around you.*

A Place For Notes:

4

Four To Eight Breathing Pattern - Stress Relief

4/8 Breathing Pattern

Bedtime breathwork or to relieve extreme stress fast.

This technique is known for its powerful effect of lowering blood pressure and decreasing the heart rate. It is an excellent practice to intentionally perform 4/8 breathing throughout the day even when not under pressure because studies show the more familiar our body is to this breathing pattern the body will naturally choose to do it because it wants the results of homeostasis (stability in the whole body). Why not make it easier when under extreme pressure to get calm NOW? So, when counting sheep to sleep doesn't work this breath pattern is for you. Getting the body out to fight and flight mode. It changes the neural pathway of the sympathetic nervous system that makes us feel anxious, overwhelmed and fearful and transitions us to the parasympathetic nervous system. A place of calm and tranquility.

I absolutely love this breathwork pattern and have found the more familiar my body is to it the quicker it responds. In fact, within two to three breaths I often find my body in a better, more relaxed state and my mood improves. I also find I naturally return to it quite often. It is a great pattern to use when your body is taxed from a hard workout or when you need stamina to keep going and you want to feel calmer in your muscular and neural system.

This breath will take 10 seconds for each breath when it is paced out properly. Feel free to set a timer for one minute and see if you can make 6 breaths happen in that one minute.

Inhale through the nose 4 count and exhale with an open mouth. MAKE SOME NOISE ON THE EXHALE. This is very important because it makes a connection to the mind, body and breath. I like to feel the air passing over the back of my throat and hitting the top of my mouth just before it passes my teeth. Some practitioners like to add a seven-count hold in the middle of the inhale and exhale. I choose not to because I really want to focus on the long exhale and find that works more adequate for me. I unconsciously pause one or two seconds between, but it is not my focus to do so. Feel free to explore what works best for you. Please resist the temptation to make the four-count inhale longer. When you first start practicing this the eight-count exhale feels long. The idea is to release as much air as you can slowly while making the "ha or wha" sound.

Here is how it is done. Inhale for four counts. Exhale for 8 counts. Counts do not equal seconds. Think about each count as a beat in music.

Nose: Inhale 1 and 2 and 3 and 4. Mouth: Exhale 1 and 2 and 3 and 4 and 5 and 6 and 7 and 8.

A Place For Notes:

5

Box Breathing Pattern - Focus

BOX BREATHING

Best for focus and stress relief.

This breathing pattern is very helpful for creating deeper focus and can really help let go of negative thoughts that continue to obnoxiously keep your mind hijacked and keep you from more meaningful activities and clarity. It reduces stress and at the same time as it calms the nervous system from flight or fight behaviors. It can improve performance when you're under pressure. Because it is increasing oxygenation, reducing muscle tension, and improving focus it is an excellent technique for athletes, especially those involved in endurance sports. It is also a great technique to practice before public speaking or performance. Because this technique requires your brain to be actively counting it can trick the mind into relaxing. Many people find it useful to manage anxiety, panic attacks and improve overall mental wellness. While practicing this technique please keep in mind soft purposeful inhales and exhales. Also remember counts do not always equal seconds, however, with this particular pattern you could set a timer and perform each inhale hold and exhale in intervals of seconds making each complete breathing cycle last 16 seconds.

Nose: Inhale for 4 counts. Hold your breath for 4 counts. Mouth: Exhale for 4 counts. Hold 4 counts.

A Place For Notes:

6

Conscious Breathing - Endurance and Relaxation

Conscious Breathing

Similar to Lamaze, yet unique to the individual. Benefits include relaxation, rest, endurance and pain reduction. It is both energizing and calming.

With conscious breathing you get to pick the pace of your breath and you get to pick the sound of your breath. I found this practice to be most useful when I am on long runs or if I have pain in the body. Conscious breathing helps distract the body, helps find a rhythm your body likes and helps balance oxygen to CO_2 rating in the body making each cycle of breath impactful for the goals stated above. This breathing pattern also has a little more force behind it. I find it most comfortable to breathe into the ribcage and chest and exhale chest, ribs cage, and belly.

Take two or three short quick inhales and one longer exhale. You may notice the exhale is about as long or just a pulse longer than the two inhales in total. Make some noise. I invite you to pick a sound for the inhale and a separate sound for the exhale. My favorite is "hu hu" for the inhale and "Hee" for the exhale.

Nose: Inhale with the sound 'hu hu'. Mouth: *Exhale "Hee"*

A Place For Notes:

BUT WHAT IF?

We talked a lot in this book about resting and relaxing, but what about when stress relief requires taking action or keeping commitments when you are tired and need to find energy? Check out these next two recommendations.

7

Lions Breath - Confidence

Lions Breath

Best for tension relief, improving circulation, energizing, improving confidence and easing the mind. It is beneficial for the neck muscles in the front of the neck. It also helps create warmth in the body.

It may feel a little silly when first learning this practice, but it has powerful benefits and is worth a deeper dive. When I first was learning this technique there was no talk about the body posture or use of hands, eyes and shoulders. What I discovered was even with just the mouth and tongue I had powerful results in relaxing muscles and tension in the head, neck and jaw. This activating breath pattern made me feel freer and more available to function in strength. So be brave and be bold because this one is a little strange at first. Let go of the socially acceptable ideals placed on us over the years and do this one for your health.

It can be practiced laying down in a relaxed position, but

traditionally it is taught on the knees with ankles crossed in back and hands on the mat with fingers pointing toward the body. This is most likely very uncomfortable if you are not a yogi. So please keep in mind what works best for you and say yes to that.

Here are some recommended positions to start with and grow into.

● Option one: Lay on back and be relaxed focusing only on the neck, head and tongue. Don't worry about the arms currently.

● Option two: Lay down on your back with knees bent and feet on the ground hip distance apart or wider. press hands into the leg just above the knees with fingers spread apart.

● Option three: Sit in a chair with legs apart on exhales, press hands into the leg just above the knees with fingers spread apart.

● Option four: Sit on your calves. Legs can be wide or together. Hands in the same position as option two.

● Option five: (Advanced) Sitting on legs with knees apart and ankles crossed over each other behind you. Hands will be placed and pressing into the floor fingers spread wide. You can also have hands on the floor with fingers pointing in the direction of your body. Press into the floor on exhales.

Pick the position option that resonates best with you at this time

and know you can choose to explore other options if you have the desire in the future.

The inhale is through the nose and the exhale happens with the mouth wide open and the tongue sticking out. Imagine how a lion yawns with its tongue wide and flat curled downward. You want to have the left and right edges of the tongue energized. So you may feel the edges of the tongue curl up and a little inward. Finally, be vocal. Make a loud long "ha" sound with the exhale. Feel the air vibrate across the back of the throat as it exits the mouth.

MOUTH WITH TONGUE STICKING OUT.
   Nose: Full inhale. Mouth: Full exhale with tongue sticking out, with the sound "hhaaaaa"

If you choose options two through five, notice hands and shoulder blades are sympathetically connected as you press into the floor or knees. Notice how the shoulder blade presses deeply down and inward into your back to help lift the heart. Imagine someones sneaks behind you and puts a cold ice cube down your shirt in between your shoulders. Surprise! That is the feeling you are looking for in shoulder placement. If you allow the shoulders to slouch forward, the activation and stretch in the chest and neck will significantly be decreased and not allow you to receive the full benefit of the lions breath.

A Place For Notes:

8

Circular Breath - Positivity and Warmth

Continuous or Circular breathing 4/4, 6/6, or 8/8 for a slower pace.

Not to be confused with circular breathing for musicians. Benefits include the release of negative energy and tension in the body. Increased motivation, increased circulation, and increased positive energy.

This practice requires you to breathe in and out at the same length without pausing between breaths. You can choose your count length according to your needs. It is often recorded that this type of breathing can be very energizing and motivating. It is good to know it can stimulate both blood flow and emotional flow. I love to practice this one when I cant control the environment temperature and I am cold. It is great at helping to quickly raise the body temperature.

Because continuous breathwork can bring your awareness to deeper subconscious thoughts or memories it is a good idea to have a plan of kindness toward yourself and to be understanding before you begin. If you need a break or a friend to talk to, plan in advance with your friend to share your experience. If you find yourself approaching a difficult emotional state STOP and switch your breath pattern to the 4/8 pattern mentioned earlier. Be sure to reassure yourself you are safe, and you are loved. It is not a bad thing if past traumas bubble up. They need to be able to exit your body. Just remember you are in control now. The situation is not the same. You are not the same. Your body may be telling you it is time to heal in that area and I would encourage you to pursue that healing with the support and supervision of a mental health therapist. That is a lot and I hope it doesn't scare you away from giving this pattern a try. It can be very helpful to keep your eye on the prize of better health, motivation, stronger immune system, empowerment, self-confidence and strength.

Start this practice in 30 second increments. Using 4/4 that should equate to five or six breaths. Each breath cycle may take four to five seconds if you use counts of four.

Nose: Fill up the chest and belly. Nose: Exhale belly chest. REPEAT CONTINUOUSLY FOR 30 SECONDS.

Bonus: *Sometimes it can make sense to meet the energy of your mind and body with your breath before taking it the other direction. For example if I am feeling hyper and I need to slow down I may choose to do the continuous breath work for a few seconds then go to box breathing and then to 4/8 technique all with in two or three minutes. This can be a really great practice to get the body to cooperate with what your mind needs most. You could also try it in reverse if you are sleepy and need to take steps into action.*

A Place For Notes:

Please Note: All these practices have more intricate options to add if you feel you want to dive deeper into your practice and understanding. But, for the purpose of keeping things simple and making the benefit to breathwork more available quickly, I choose to leave details such as mudras for fingers, where to place the tongue, or what to do with your eyes out. The details I left out can add to your experience, but they are not required for a successful practice.

Remember once again this is a practice. The goal is progress not perfection. It does not need to be perfect. It only needs to have your attention as you rehearse and begin to understand when to apply the breathwork and which ones work best for you. I recommend practicing as much as you can in a variety of situations to help the body recognize how powerful the breath is and strengthen the natural ability to go to it with less efforts.

For your convenience I have listed below two other interesting

styles of breathwork that require deeper understanding and offer huge benefits. Because of the intense nature of these patterns, I will not be sharing the how to in this book, but rather encourage you to take a deeper look into them. Please remember to check with your medical team when you are exploring these powerful practices.

1. **Wim Hof** Created by a Dutch extreme athlete who is also known as the "Ice Man". Students are trained to use breathing techniques, cold therapy, and commitment.

Benefits may include immunity, better sleep, reduced stress, heightened focus, and control of the body's functions through the mind. I feel this is a great technique if you are interested in learning more of a mind over matter practice.

1. **Holotropic (to move in the direction of something) Breathwork** Created by Stanislav Grof, MD, and his late wife Christina.

Benefits may include promoting the release of toxins from your bloodstream and tissue. Lowering blood pressure by increasing circulation. Boost immune system. Improve digestion. Reduce stress on the liver and kidneys. Reduce physical and emotional stress. Increase clarity and creativity, create new neural pathways in the brain. When practiced with a mental health specialist. It can be used to help support the individual suffering from depression, substance use disorder, post-traumatic stress disorder, anxiety, negative thinking, chronic stress, tension, and avoidance behaviors.

9

Things you may experience

Breathwork can have so many positive effects and everyone's experience can vary immensely. It can offer calm and peace, but it can also be intense. You might feel light, warm, heavy and anchored into the ground. You may feel tingling all over or you may feel muscular sensations releasing tension patterns similar to rolling, pulsing, or vibrations. You may also discover deep emotional releases and freedom from pain. Some may cry or scream or begin shaking with the intention to let the energy move through and out of the body. Some may feel so at peace they fall asleep. While at other times they feel the need to put on their tennis shoes and run. It can be enlightening and make it feel as if all the questions of the world have easy to access answers or even feel like an out of body experience with an altered state of consciousness. You may feel super creative or inspired. You may see color or feel sensations throughout the body that have no rhyme or reason. Whatever you might experience it is all normal and your personal experience. It is all with a purpose that doesn't need to even make sense. Just know this is your journey, your experience and there is no right or wrong. Always feel free to take a moment and note how you feel and things you notice in your body and thoughts. Keep in mind that may not even mean writing words. You may prefer to draw, paint, sing, dance or build something. What ever you decide to do feel completely free to express yourself. If you feel safe you may even like to video record your experience and the expression of it for future personal exploration.

10

Suggestions of combinations to get you started.

Pick your goal and give the recommended sequence a try.

Peace and Calm

Lay down in a comfortable position. If you can not lay down, sit down. If sitting is not an option that's okay too. But always choose to lay down if that is an option.

Sound can be set to 396 Hz, 528 Hz, or 432 Hz. Simply google search Music set to ... Apple, Spotify, and YouTube all have these types of categories.

Set the colors of the room to Blue or Green shades. This can be lighting or a pillow and a blanket. If this is not an option imagine the blue sky, blue water, tops of trees or the grass.

Close your eyes if that is an option. If you are not in a place you can close your eyes try to focus on one object and relax the gaze around that one object.

Choose to imagine yourself in your favorite place. Imagine Smelling your favorite smell. Imagine tasting your favorite taste. Touch you fingers together and feel your presence.

Begin to practice the **Three Part Breath** and continue to ground yourself

If you can really take the time to relax switch to **4/8 Breathing** pattern when you are feeling grounded from the three part breath.

Focus

Sit down. If sitting is not an option that's okay to. But always choose to sit if that is an option.

Sound can be set to 852 Hz, 528 Hz, or 432 Hz. Simply google search Music set to... Apple, Spotify, and YouTube all have these types of categories.

Set the colors of the room to Red, Yellow or Blue shades. This can be lighting or even an object or photograph. If it is not an option to have special lighting or objects of specific colors look at a photo of the color on your phone or imagine the a bright sunny day, the red rock canons, or flowing water.

Close your eyes if that is an option.

Rub your hands on your legs in a small circle or cross your arms and touch opposite shoulders. Feel free to tap.

Choose to imagine yourself in your favorite place or with a person you feel is inspiring.

Begin to practice **Box Breathing.**

Feel free to practice **Lions Breath** first if you are feeling anxious.

Energizing

Sitting or standing.

Sound can be set to 741 Hz, 417 Hz, or 432 Hz. Simply google search Music set to ... Apple, Spotify, and YouTube all have these types of categories.

Set the colors of the room to Red, Orange, or Yellow shades. This can be lighting or if that is not an option imagine Running and winning a race, Hopping up and down with excitement or your favorite thing in any of those colors.

Blink your eyes as fast as you can for a moment or two. Bring your attention to the back of your eyes fading out the details in front of you. Now blinking normally.

Begin to practice **Consistent/Circular Breath**.

If you are having a hard time starting, zero in on **Box Breathing** first. Then take it to **Consistent Breath** practice when you are ready.

Wisdom/Understanding

Take any position or posture you are comfortable in.

Sound can be set to 964 Hz, 528 Hz, or 852. Simply google search Music set to ... Apple, Spotify, and YouTube all have these types of categories.

Set the colors of the room to Violet or Indigo shades. This can be lighting or if that is not an option surround yourself with objects of that color. Or you may choose to think of a favorite thing in any of those colors.

Relax and soften your gaze or close your eyes

Feel free to make a tiny circle between the eyes, Tap the heart zone, or tap the top of the head for a moment. Just to wake up circulation in those areas.

Begin to practice **Lions Breath.**

If you are having a hard time starting focus on **Box Breathing** first.

11

Conclusion

In conclusion I would like to take a moment to congratulate you on taking up breathwork and not giving up on this practice even when it has been difficult in the past. You can do it and you can feel successful as long as you remember it's okay to be human. It's okay to make mistakes and its about making progress no matter how big or little at a time that progress happens. You do get to have control over your body, and mind. Breathwork is work and it does take time, practice, and commitment to get better at it. Pick one pattern and just practice that pattern until you feel like it makes sense in your body and is easy to do. Revisit it often and play with the idea of trying it in different situations or positions like standing up, sitting down or laying down. You have this handy little book to reflect on if you ever feel like trying a different pattern for a different circumstance. When you are ready explore the suggested combinations in the last chapter and maybe even make your own. Take your time and never feel pressured to be perfect according to what works for someone else. Your experience is uniquely and perfectly yours. Remember you already are breathing and now you have some tools to make that breath support you in each moment day and night. You got this and I believe in you.

If you have learned something from this book or feel this book has helped you, I hope you will leave a favorable review on amazon and recommend it to your friends. One breath at a time, we can make a difference in each of our lives. Thank you so much for sharing.

Resources

mindbodygreen. (2022, July 7). *The incredible power of the breath & how to tap into it on demand.* Mindbodygreen. https://www.mindbodygreen.com/articles/what-breathwork-is

Nash, J., PhD. (2024, May 23). *7 best breathwork Techniques & Exercises to use.* PositivePsychology.com. https://positivepsychology.com/breathwork-techniques/

Breathwork for beginners: What to know and how to get started. (2024, April 30). Cleveland Clinic. https://health.clevelandclinic.org/breathwork

Elmer, J. (2022, June 10). *Anxiety can cause shortness of breath And what you can do.* Healthline. https://www.healthline.com/health/shortness-of-breath-anxiety#symptoms

Harmonance | Sound Healing Frequencies | Wellness Soundscapes. (n.d.). https://www.harmonance.com/

Llc, B. (2020, December 9). Colored Light Effects: How they Impact your body and mood. *BlissLights.* https://blisslights.com/blogs/blisslights/colored-light-effects-how-they-impact-your-body-and-mood

www.ingramcontent.com/pod-product-compliance
Lightning Source LLC
Chambersburg PA
CBHW072341270726
48659CB00023B/2170